Toward Better Behavior: Yours, Mine, and Everyone Else's

A Strategy for Improving the Assessment and Long-Term Care Planning Process

Barbara F. Speedling

© 2017 Barbara F. Speedling
All rights reserved.

ISBN: 1979333785
ISBN-13: 9781979333788

What Keeps Us from Better Behavior?

"When you don't get what you want, you get an attitude."
-Regina, (57), Brooklyn, NY
Nursing Home Resident

With Gratitude

Thank you to all the elders and individuals with disabilities who have shared thoughts and feelings with me. It is through their generosity that I can share the insights that follow.

Foreword

Barbara Speedling and I first met due to our shared love of music. She had founded a nonprofit music school in Flushing, New York called CenterStage. I became a board member.

Barbara had studied voice as a young lady and wanted to make music available to both children and adults in the community; I had begun piano lessons at age six and, as a medical student, helped support myself by performing solo piano in bars and restaurants in Bern, Switzerland which is where I studied to become a physician.

We soon realized that we had another common interest. Barbara was engaged nationwide in providing her expertise in the care of nursing home patients. She lectured at many institutions and was highly regarded in the field; I had served for three years early in my career as a house physician at a large county-operated nursing home in Uniondale, New York. We found we had much to talk about besides arranging music lessons for large numbers of students.

One of my colleagues at that nursing home, a prominent physician who remains my most beloved mentor, truly revolutionized care in the facility. He was a Holocaust survivor and a man who loved, indeed, savored life.

Because he knew that the worst part of aging is a loss of purpose, he was determined to give our patients more than first-rate medical care – he wanted to ensure they had a reason to go on living. Women were encouraged to prepare food in the facility kitchens for visiting relatives; men were taken by bus to the fishing pier at Jones Beach for outings. All patients were invited and taken by bus on different mornings to the live performances of the Ray Heatherton show at Roosevelt Raceway. Most importantly, all patients were urged to participate in their care.

Barbara is from the same school of thought. Her first book, *Why is Grandma Screaming?*, touches thoughtfully on the challenges of caring for the demented elderly among us. This book is a follow up, giving even more information on how to better relate to this group of mentally compromised patients. The ways she interacts with demented patients are insightful and instructive. I believe both books should be required reading for health care providers, as they are being trained to care for patients with complex behavioral health needs.

Training health care providers to deal with elderly demented patients, and others with special needs, is a major and universal health care problem. Providing humane care can be exceedingly frustrating since patients are frequently uncooperative or non-compliant. They often cannot be counted on to follow staff instructions. As staff members lose patience there is an increase in the potential for elder abuse.

Barbara has developed remarkable insights in how to best address this problem. When staff follows her practices, patients are often more cooperative and comfortable. Caregivers find themselves better satisfied in their duties.

Barbara prepared herself for her career in patient care through both academic study and hands-on interaction. While studying music in college, she worked as a driver and attendant for a disability transportation service on campus. She credits this experience with shaping the foundation of her perspective on quality of life.

Barbara devotes this second book to instructions on how to assess patients: how to develop an understanding of how and why they are uncooperative, and how best to communicate with them in a positive way. The book contains many examples of the way her techniques can control a variety of stressful situations to the benefit of both the patients and staff.

As I have personally experienced the caregiving problems to which she has dedicated herself, and having attended a lecture she gave to members of the health care community, I am certain this book will contribute to a significant improvement in one of the most vexing problems facing our country: the safe, compassionate, stimulating care of our elderly and demented.

Donald Margouleff, M.D. FACP

Learning the Difference between Behavior and Response
An Introduction

I've spent the better part of my career in long-term care observing and interviewing people others find challenging. In most cases, what is described to me as *behavior* is often a common-place reaction to something that is happening to the person. Here are some examples:

- In the case of Alzheimer's dementia, the wandering behavior I am asked to address is a symptom of the illness. There are a limited number of things that might make the person stop moving, such as offering food or an engaging activity, but both would be short-lived diversions for the person who is experiencing psychomotor agitation[1]. The most practical intervention for wandering behavior is to make it as safe as possible for the person to satisfy the need to move. In other words, accommodating the behavior is the most effective way of ensuring that intervention is therapeutic and person-centered.
- A person diagnosed with paranoia responds poorly to an inventory of personal belongings conducted in his or her absence by a staff member. Avoiding this negative reaction requires an understanding of the disease and an anticipation of what might happen in such a scenario. To accommodate this behavior, consider allowing the person to participate in the inventory process. Doing so minimizes the potential for accusations

---

1 Niedens, L.S.C.S.W., Michelle. "The Neuropsychiatric Symptoms of Dementia." Alz.org, **https://www.alz.org/documents/heartofamerica/Neuropsych_Book_LR.pdf**. (Accessed July 10, 2017)

of theft or damage to the person's belongings, and offers an opportunity for collaboration with the caregiver(s).
- There are times when the challenging behavior is simply an aspect of an individual's personality. A person who is outspoken might be described as having too many opinions. Someone who is used to being in control might be described as demanding. Those who refuse to abide by institutional schedules may be said to be non-compliant. In cases such as these, when the challenge is personality driven, it becomes even more important to adopt the holistic approach to assessment I describe later in this book.

The advent of new federal behavioral health regulatory language adopted in 2016, the mandate for considering pharmacologic intervention alternatives, requires a closer look at what is meant by person-centered care. As the long-term care demographics continue to shift and diversify, the greater the need to understand people as individuals. Achieving such understanding presents new challenges and considerations in assessment and care planning.

This book is the first in a series of discussions about individuals I've had the pleasure to know in a variety of long-term care settings. Each case illustrates the importance of distinguishing the differences among symptoms of illness, reactions to circumstances, and individual resident personality in evaluating and responding to behavioral health needs.

Exploring the realities of institutional living, as well as its impact on mood and behavior and quality of life, was the subject of my first book, *Why is Grandma Screaming?* While long-term care facilities once cared almost exclusively for the frail elderly, many of whom had also been diagnosed with dementia, today's populations are far more varied in age, disability, and psychosocial circumstances. That makes understanding "what makes someone tick" more complicated, at best.

In this book, I hope to inspire professional caregivers to look more closely at the people they serve and to come to a deeper understanding of what motivates people to do what they do. Doing so begins with recognizing the similarities between your behavior and the behavior of the person who presents you with a challenge.

After reading this book, ask yourself two questions: given the same set of circumstances, do you think your behavior would be very different from that of the person you are trying to figure out? And, what would it take to satisfy your needs in the same situation?

I think you'll find it is the logical place to begin your journey to improved assessment.

one

Learning to Accommodate Behavior: Yours, Mine, and Everyone Else's

Learning to accommodate behavior, yours, mine, and everyone else's, is an increasingly important social skill as Americans become ever more diverse along political, economic, racial, and ethnic lines. Nowhere is it more important than within the context of long-term care.

Behavior is defined by Webster's as "the way someone conducts themselves."[2] There is a second definition, one indicating that some behavior is in response to an individual's environment. That definition would include reactions to behavior of others in the environment.

For example, when I have been confronted by a server in a restaurant who has been less than courteous, I have sometimes reacted by being less than courteous in return. Or, when forced to share a public space with a noisy person, I might show agitation. My mood can be influenced by the mood and behavior of those around me.

The way I express my mood may be different from the way others do. If I am crying, I am frustrated, not sad. If I am quiet, perhaps I'm angry. How will you know what I am communicating if you never ask how I express my emotions?

The first step to understanding and accommodating behavior is to know what is normal for the individual. Questions routinely found on assessment documents pay little attention to personality, occupation, habits, or lifestyle.

---

2 **https://www.merriam-webster.com/dictionary/behavior** (Accessed June 27, 2017)

Consider the gentleman newly admitted to the nursing home following a stroke. He can no longer express himself. The assigned caregiver assists him with his personal care, which includes helping him put on his pajamas.

As she does this he resists her. She tries to put the pajama top on; he attempts to pull the pajama top off. This goes on for several minutes until he is tired and resists no more. The pajamas are put on successfully… and removed ten minutes later by the resident.

After several nights of the pajama war, the attending physician is called and a psychiatric evaluation is ordered to assess the resident's behavior. The psychiatric evaluation determines the resident has stroke-related anxiety and that this may be the cause of his restless, stripping behavior. An anti-anxiety medication is ordered to address the behavior.

Despite medication, the resident continues to remove his pajamas. The care plan team meets and revises the plan: he will sleep in a gown instead of pajamas. No luck. He removes the gown as well.

At last resort, the team purchases pajamas designed to prevent unwanted removal. This makes the resident angry. He becomes more restless and agitated than before. His reaction reaches near-violence. As a result, the care plan team contacts the resident's daughter, who is his healthcare agent, and convenes a meeting about this behavior.

The daughter reveals that her father has always slept naked. The question was never asked during assessment. Consequently, this preference and long-standing habit was unknown, leading the care team to see it as something abnormal. Rather than consider that the resident's initial resistance could be an attempt to communicate that pajamas were not part of his routine the caregivers immediately saw the resistance as non-compliance.

There are several ways the team could have improved this situation:

1) it could have revised the assessment process to include more questions specific to the person's usual routine and preferred way of doing things;

2) it could have asked the resident's daughter about her father's personal preferences, including sleep habits, at the time of admission; and

3) it could have notified the resident's daughter following the first resistance episode so that it would have had more insight into her father's behavior before the situation escalated.

Had one or more of these things been implemented, this *behavior* may never have occurred. Looking more deeply at the individual's life before he or she was admitted, as well as considering the traumatic shift from that life to an institutional life, is an effective way to understand and, in many cases, anticipate and accommodate the moods and reactions that may play out in the caregiving environment.

It is also possible to anticipate some behavior based on what is known about the resident's previous lifestyle or his or her ethnicity.

For example, a resident born in the American patriarchal society of the 1920's is more likely to follow the instructions of a male caregiver than that of a female caregiver. In that case, generational orientation may have an impact on the way a person responds to others.

On the other hand, here is how ethnicity can have an impact. A resident of Chinese descent will generally not make eye-contact when being introduced. For the Chinese, it is considered impolite to stare into another's eyes. By comparison, a resident of Latin descent will expect eye-contact and a strong handshake.[3] Understanding cultural habits is another vital piece of mood and behavior assessment because long-term care populations are increasingly diverse.

The second step in interpreting a person's behavior is understanding how the disease process, or the circumstances leading up to such chronic conditions as alcoholism or opioid addiction, have

---

3 Country Guides: China. commisceo-global.com. **http://www.commisceo-global.com/country-guides**/. (Accessed January 7, 2017)

an impact on the person's mood and behavior. The person who sustains a spinal cord injury while high on cocaine may have always indulged in risky behavior. It could be a symptom of undiagnosed and untreated bipolar disorder. By identifying the motivation for the risk-taking behavior, and the resulting substance use, better behavior assessment and appropriate intervention is possible.

Another example of the way disease has an impact on behavior is in the person who develops Alzheimer's disease and exhibits agitated, aggressive behavior uncharacteristic of his or her pre-dementia personality. As the disease results in diminished social filters and the ability to control impulsive behavior, it is reasonable to anticipate that agitation or aggressive behavior will be the response to situations that the individual finds incomprehensible. While such behavior would never be exhibited before the diagnosis, it is now something over which the person has little control.

The third and final step in this process of understanding behavior is personality assessment. It includes gathering details as to how the person previously lived and responded to the world. This is the most difficult and the most helpful piece of the puzzle.

Take the business owner who worked long hours and sacrificed time with his family and friends because he wanted to leave a financially secure legacy for his children. He now finds himself living among strangers in an assisted living facility. His children have long since sold the business and the family home, and all have gone their separate ways. The few friends he once had have passed away. He is angry, disappointed, bored, and lonely.

He is described by caregivers as impatient, rude, and unfriendly toward others living in the community. Considering his lifestyle and the description of his workaholic personality, the caregivers should anticipate that this is a man who has difficulty taking direction, who needs to be busy and productive, and who has little experience at socializing with strangers.

Once they understand his emotional circumstances, both of loneliness and his disappointment in his children, it may also lead the caregivers to anticipating symptoms of depression. All too often depression manifests as anger, irritability, or withdrawal,[4] leading caregivers to misinterpret the behavior as something other than a symptom of illness.

A behavioral health plan for this man might involve an assessment and intervention for depression; development of a personality profile to help caregivers become more familiar with the individual, his occupation, and his lifestyle; development of a therapeutic activity structure to support his need to be engaged and productive, and opportunities for socialization in small, non-threatening groups.

This last item, accommodating his limited social experience by allowing him to ease into social situations, may result in a more positive reaction than if he were expected to be comfortable sitting in a dayroom amid a large group of strangers.

While many assessment tools are used in long-term care, few include the kinds of questions necessary for identifying factors and circumstances that influence an individual's mood and behavior. Two people with wandering behavior may have very different motivations for moving and searching. By identifying and understanding the differences, the resulting interventions become more person-centered.

For example, one person's motivation for moving and searching may merely be a manifestation of the psychomotor agitation common to an Alzheimer's dementia diagnosis.[5] In this case, a successful intervention would include creating a safe place for wandering and rummaging. Doing so not only accommodates the symptom, but also minimizes the risk of altercations since it reduces the need to wander in on others.

Another person's moving and searching motivation may be based in the delusion that she is a prisoner and secret notes from her husband

---

[4] National Institute of Mental Health. "Depression: Overview." nimh.nih.gov. **https://www.nimh.nih.gov/health/topics/depression/index.shtml#part_145397**. (Accessed July 10, 2017)

[5] Niedens, L.S.C.S.W., Michelle. "The Neuropsychiatric Symptoms of Dementia." Alz.org, **https://www.alz.org/documents/heartofamerica/Neuropsych_Book_LR.pdf**. (Accessed July 10, 2017)

are hidden in various places in the prison. Delusions are a common symptom of schizophrenia, particularly if the disease is not well-managed. A successful intervention for this individual would include developing a comprehensive plan addressing her mental health needs. Such a plan would likely include individual psychotherapy and therapeutic diversionary activity.

In this case, by appropriately addressing the disease through psychotherapy or pharmacologic intervention or a combination of the two, a diversionary plan can also be developed to support the resident's orientation. Activities reinforcing current date and circumstance, such as reading the newspaper together or looking at photographs of the person's life in a chronological display, may diminish delusional behavior by supplementing the other treatments.

Other important aspects of assessment should include the way a person typically expressed extreme emotion pre-diagnosis. Was there yelling, cursing, striking out, or other signs of agitation or aggression? Following those episodes of extreme emotion what was the self-soothing technique? In my practice, I can think of many cases in which I've been involved where challenging behavior was consistent with the way the pre-dementia or pre-illness/disability personality was described by family or other close friends or associates. The caregivers evaluating it simply didn't know or understand the behavior for what it was.

When I am in session with caregivers I often ask them how they personally express anger and how they soothe themselves afterwards. The answers are as varied as the people in the room.

Some report yelling, cursing, or just being extremely loud. Others say they are silent and withdraw from the situation. Still others slam objects or throw them, or strike out physically.

As important as it is to understand how people express emotion, it is equally important to understand how they help themselves calm down. Again, some caregivers in my sessions report they go shopping after they become angry or frustrated, or when weighing a complicated situation or decision. Others said they go for a walk and it is the physical activity that helps them vent the energy which can follow an episode of extreme emotion. Eating is also a popular response, as is indulging in alcohol or smoking marijuana. Risk-taking behaviors are also reported, such as gambling or fast driving. For others, a warm bath and a good night's rest are helpful, as is a soothing massage. Whatever the remedy, few of the options the caregivers personally use can be accessed or practiced in a long-term care environment.

Consider, for example, the elderly woman accustomed to rising early each day and going to the local park to take her morning walk. Following a stroke, she continues to want to do what she has always done. She wakes early, before dawn, and attempts to get out of bed, just as she has done all her life. Only now, she is unable to stand or walk without assistance. She doesn't realize this and tries to stand on her own. She falls. She repeats the attempt daily and each day she falls.

Her caregivers are at a loss to understand this *behavior*. They never consider that this once may have been a productive or habitual ritual, only one that now sadly results in her repeated failure to stand and the inevitable fall to the floor. Had the caregiving team considered her age (she is a *Baby Boomer*); the typical lifestyle of a woman of her background (she held a management position at a women's wellness center, she is a vegetarian and she meditates); and analyzed the pattern of the falls, it may not have considered her actions as *behavior*. Instead, the team may have entertained the possibility that she was an early riser who once started her day at the gym or with some other form of physical activity. Considering her actions from this perspective, and not just categorizing her as someone who is "non-compliant with call bell use," opens a whole new realm of care plan reasoning and possibilities.

Occupation, position, ethnicity, social status, and domestic and leisure routines are all important in understanding who the person was and is, and in anticipating habits and reactions to the current circumstances. The roles such factors play in a successful assessment are often overlooked when the situation is complicated by a neurodegenerative disease, such as dementia, Parkinson's disease, or multiple sclerosis, or by a mental disorder such as schizophrenia or bipolar disorder. Isolating the challenging behavior as solely a symptom of one or more of these diseases may lead caregivers to misunderstand and mislabel what was once understood as *normal* for this person.

If families or friends who are close to the resident are to be the source of information about pre-diagnosis status or behavior, it is important to conduct a non-threatening admissions interview. Otherwise, family and friends are likely to feel uncomfortable in divulging what may be perceived as the family's dirty laundry. They may be reluctant or simply refuse to share intimate details of personal behavior that may or may not include alcoholism, domestic violence, elder abuse, criminal history, or other trauma.

If not sensitively and carefully elicited during the admissions interview, such challenges will eventually surface after admission when they will be too slowly addressed through the care plan process.

Knowing what to ask in an interview is just one important aspect of successful assessment. Knowing who, when, and where to interview are equally important in obtaining as much accurate information as possible. The next chapter explains how to develop an interviewing approach that is more social than clinical so that residents, families, and close friends feel comfortable sharing information that improves outcomes.

two

Improving the Interview Process

I recently conducted an interview at a man's bedside. He was newly admitted to a nursing home and he had a dementia diagnosis. Our conversation was interrupted several times as he leaned in to kiss me. Each time, I politely reminded him who I was and why I was there. He would nod, say he understood, and sit back in his chair – only to attempt to kiss me again in a few minutes.

I realized afterward that I should not have been surprised about his confusion as to the nature of my visit. After all, we were in his bedroom and kissing often occurs in a bedroom. Affected by memory loss, he most likely assumed I was in his bedroom for something other than an interview. Based on this experience, I now rarely interview anyone in the bedroom. I've also learned over the years that location is just one of many factors that can mean the difference between a productive and unproductive interview.

Planning the Interview

A person newly admitted to either a day program or a residential placement should be given time to adjust to the move's trauma before extensive interviews begin. The admitting team should focus on helping the person settle in and feel comfortable with the new circumstances before collecting information. Much of what is initially needed can be found in the documents that either preceded or accompanied the person.

Before approaching someone I am going to interview, I first like to observe. How does he occupy himself? How does she interact with others? If observation is done during meals or activity programs there is the added advantage of insight into social behavior and functional ability.

Sometimes the person may be in a later stage of dementia and unable to respond in a conversational interview. When that's the case, observation becomes vital to identifying potential interventions for the common challenges of wandering, rummaging, or inappropriate social or sexual behavior.

My preference is to review medical records or interview the caregiving team after I interview the resident. That way, I approach the initial interview without prejudice. The information in admission records or in caregiver documentation is often subjective.

For example, while one caregiver may ascribe agitation or aggression to an episode in which the person used a raised voice, another team member might have simply recognized the episode as a natural, common-place response for anyone whose frustration is allowed to escalate.

Since the interview process leads to the initial care profile, information from which is then incorporated into the comprehensive assessment and care plan, it is important to plan the interview carefully.

Conducting the Interview

In November 2016, the Centers for Medicare and Medicaid Services (CMS) published *Final Rules for Participation*. The rules outline the revised federal regulations and standards for long-term care facilities if they are to remain eligible for Medicare and Medicaid funding.

Long-term care facilities are now required to complete an interdisciplinary, baseline care plan within forty-eight hours of admission.[6] For that reason, it is more important than ever to streamline the new admission interview process.

---

6 Centers for Medicare and Medicaid, State Operations Manual, Appendix PP. F655, §483.21(a) Baseline Care Plans

To help my clients improve the admission interview experience, I've recommended they establish a welcome process. This process ensures that the primary Certified Nursing Assistant (CNA) is the person who greets the new resident, orients them to the environment, and initiates the interview process. This approach improves the relationship between the primary caregiver and the resident, prevents the need to overwhelm the new resident with many different interviews, and minimizes the potential for a negative first impression. Moreover, information about personal preferences, routines, and lifestyle choices will be obtained by the person who, more than anyone else, needs to know how to achieve person-centered, person-directed care.

It is common for new residents with a dementia diagnosis or similar cognitive deficit to react poorly to nursing home admission. Moving to a nursing home is something no one plans to do, no one is ever very happy about, and the potential for elopement is real.

In the long-term care world "elopement" is not a prelude to a romantic adventure. Quite the contrary, it is a euphemism for "escape," a high-risk episode for any resident but even more dangerous for someone with dementia or a similar condition. To minimize the danger, long-term care environments generally employ an alarm system. It alerts the staff either to the attempt or actual elopement by someone in their care, and it's a system I do not favor.

Such a system sounds an audible alarm each time a resident moves too close to a sensor location. Imagine your own irritation in being monitored in this fashion, setting off an alarm any time you venture too close to an entrance or exit. For people with a dementia diagnosis who may already believe they are being held captive by strangers, these alarms are more than irritating. They are frightening and they complicate an already difficult and dangerous situation.

I recommend, instead, allowing the primary caregiver to develop, through the initial admission interview, a relationship with the resident that fosters trust and familiarity. Both are essential to helping a resident calmly accept the need for intimate care and in reducing the fear that prompts flight.

The initial interview should start by gathering information necessary to the development of the baseline care plan, such as diagnosis, treatment and medication orders, and food allergies. After that, there is time to obtain social history, behavioral health needs, and other personal information.

Questions about specific aspects of former lifestyles should be included, such as what is normally worn to bed or what was the former daytime routine. The stripping behavior I described in the earlier section is not unique to that individual, which is why I stress the need for this information. It's a good example of how learning one small detail – that someone prefers to sleep naked – can reduce conflict through a more relevant care plan.

Other interview questions should focus on the resident's feelings about the placement, and opinions about communal living and being dependent on others. Also, as explained in the earlier chapter, learning how someone expresses anger or frustration is an important part of understanding and anticipating behavioral health needs. Questions about that, and questions that identify how the person has always calmed anger or frustration, should be included in the interview process.

Now that the federal government has issued new regulations for Trauma Informed Care[7], the treatment framework that involves understanding, recognizing and responding to the effects of all types of trauma, delving more deeply into the person's psychosocial history and life events is essential to understanding the individual's unique needs. While the most well-known, there is trauma other than the Post Traumatic Stress Disorder (PTSD) most often associated with combat veterans. Trauma may stem from a motor vehicle accident, a house fire, a robbery, a miscarriage, domestic violence, and, yes, giving up your life and everything you've worked for to move to a nursing home.

---

7 Centers for Medicare and Medicaid, State Operations Manual, Appendix PP. F699 §483.25(m) Trauma-informed care.

Identifying trauma, and its role in creating behavioral health needs, helps the caregiving team more clearly identify how both clinical and social circumstances have had an impact on the individual. It is key information that can result in a more personalized and meaningful care plan.

Where an interview is conducted is critical to the outcome. For most people, the preferred location would be a private, quiet place, devoid of excessive noise or distraction. Unfortunately, new participant interviews at adult day health centers, or at residential or skilled facilities, are too often conducted in an area that diminishes the person's ability to concentrate and communicate.

Overcoming sensory and communication deficits is another great challenge in the interview process. If a resident normally wears eyeglasses or hearing aids, be sure they are in place before the interview begins. Pictures or word cues, or a computer-based communication program, facilitates the interview process. When I interview, I often bring up pictures stored on my smart phone because it helps the person grasp the details of our conversation.

Facial expression and body language are important to setting the tone of the interview. Most people greeted by someone who is smiling will smile in return. Someone in the later stages of dementia, or someone who has a hearing loss, responds first to facial expression. Approaching a resident with a smile paves the way for a more comfortable exchange.

The tone or volume of your voice is important. For example, someone who has suffered a stroke or who has an Alzheimer's disease diagnosis may also have a speech language disorder known as aphasia.[8] Someone with aphasia will respond first to the tone and volume of your voice because your words may not be understood.

---

8 *Aphasia* is a communication disorder that results from damage to the parts of the brain that contain language. Aphasia may cause difficulties in speaking, listening, reading, and writing, but does not affect intelligence. American Speech Language Hearing Association. ASHA.org.

http://www.asha.org/public/speech/disorders/Aphasia/ (Accessed June 16 2017)

Offering your hand, as opposed to taking the other person's hand, is another non-threatening way to greet someone. There are those who prefer not to shake hands and some for whom shaking hands is not a cultural custom. For those with a mental disorder, shaking hands or being touched by a stranger may be perceived as unsanitary or threatening.

If you offer your hand and the person does not accept your gesture, move on. This should be your first observation of how the person behaves in new or unfamiliar circumstances. The interaction is likely to change as the person becomes comfortable with you and the interview. Keep in mind that it may take several interviews over a week or several weeks to develop a true picture of the person and what he or she needs to thrive.

Adjust your position so that you make eye contact. Be sure that area lighting is sufficient for those with impaired vision. Remember that people in later stages of Alzheimer's disease develop tunnel vision and other perceptual deficits.[9] For the interview to be successful, you must be alert to and ready to accommodate such vision challenges.

Conducting a conversational interview, as opposed to a question-and-answer session, helps people feel more comfortable.

When I interview, I adopt an informal demeanor and refrain from taking copious notes. Instead, I remember the important details and document them after the interview.

It can occasionally be helpful to share a personal experience that mirrors the individual's experience. For example, I genuinely empathize with those who have lost a loved one to suicide because I have experienced that pain. I shared that in an interview with a young woman who had witnessed a friend's overdose-related suicide. She believed I understood her feelings because I had lived through something similar. Our common experience differentiated me from

---

9 Larkin, Carole. "Tunnel Vision in Alzheimer's and Related Dementia." Alzheimer's Reading Room. Alz.org.

http://www.alzheimersreadingroom.com/2012/12/tunnel-vision-in-alzheimers-and-related.html (Accessed July 10, 2017) the many other professionals to whom she had told her story, and it made for a more open conversation.

Some health care professionals discourage such an exchange and their reservations have merit. Used judiciously, however, it can elicit information critical to the overall goal: the most effective personalized care plan.

As addiction and substance use has become more widespread among long-term care populations, it is another important reason to clearly identify the circumstances underlying challenging behavior.

Here is a good example: I interviewed a young man admitted to a nursing home directly from the local prison. A double-amputee, he required skilled nursing services for wound care, services which were unavailable in prison. He sustained his injury in a drive-by shooting resulting from gang activity. He admits he is a "pothead" and has, of late, been using methamphetamine.

Since admission he frightens his elderly neighbors by yelling at them, playing loud music, or pushing them from behind. He insults the staff, and often makes comments and gestures toward female staff that are sexual in nature. One time, he drove his motorized wheelchair over an elderly man's toes causing him to fall and sustain injury. His motivation? The older man was "moving too slowly." He is regularly demanding, vulgar in conversation, and socially off-putting. He is prone to obscene action during personal care,

The threats of the caregiving team to discharge him if his behavior does not improve have no impact on him. During our interview, he told me he didn't want to be in the nursing home, so if behaving badly would get him "out of this hellhole," that was fine with him.

His lack of concern or consideration for the staff or other residents should have been anticipated. Given the lifestyle information available pre-admission, it was naïve of the caregivers to expect him to have concern for the feelings or well-being of others.

At a minimum, the team must ask itself three questions: what type of person becomes a gang member? What does that lifestyle suggest about the resident's education, social development, and general sense of self-worth? Why did the resident turn to drugs?

In this case, healing some of his underlying problems must come first. He must learn the importance of trust, accountability, respect, and self-esteem. These values, typically taught at home, must now be taught in his new environment, the nursing home. That paves the way to addressing the behaviors, such as drug use, which result from the lack of such values. It must be the priority of the behavioral care plan so that it becomes sustainable.

I'm often told there is not enough time or human resources to conduct an interview in the way I've described, but consider this: investing an hour of CNA time at admission, and the subsequent hour or less other disciplines spend in the initial interview process, saves the caregiving team countless fruitless hours trying to figure out why people do what they do and what can be done about it.

In the chapters that follow, I present cases in which the information I obtained through a comprehensive, holistic interview process became the foundation for a successful, person-centered plan for both clinical and psychosocial well-being. For privacy reasons, names were changed and the exact details are obscured. Even so, it's readily apparent that while the diagnoses and circumstances are different for each case, the outcome is the same.

three

Cindy

The Individual:

Cindy (41) has the following diagnoses: traumatic brain injury (TBI) secondary to heroin overdose, cardiovascular accident (CVA), multiple sclerosis (MS), bipolar depression, and anxiety disorder.

The Challenging Behavior:

Cindy is described by staff as difficult, resisting care routines and making excessive demands for attention. She is also said to be foul-mouthed, inconsiderate and abusive to her peers, and manipulative. Staff members also claim she is a hoarder.

The History:

As a child, Cindy lived with alcoholic parents who also used drugs. She endured physical abuse and later, as a teen bride, she was a victim of domestic violence.

She is divorced now and she has four biological children, all of whom are adults. Two of the children are in regular contact with her; the other two were removed from her home at a young age, placed in foster care, and eventually adopted by other families. She was estranged from the adopted children for a time, but has recently reconnected with them.

She currently has a significant other who was once a resident of the nursing home. He now lives in the community. He has traumatic brain injury and is unable to work. He visits her, as do two of her children.

The Current Situation:

After two unsuccessful discharges into the community, this is Cindy's third admission to the same nursing home. It is a small facility with a single common room serving as both dining room and dayroom. There are outdoor areas, and residents must be supervised to enjoy them. Cindy is living in a room with three additional beds, each occupied by a woman who is twice her age and who has a dementia diagnosis.

Cindy is obsessed with discharge, and devotes most of her time to searching for housing in the community and visiting with her boyfriend. She rarely attends any structured activity programs and has few social interactions with other residents. A smoker, she attends each of three supervised smoking sessions scheduled daily, which take place outside.

The Assessment:

I find Cindy in her room. She has fashioned a cocoon for herself by pulling the privacy curtains together to completely envelop her bed. I call to her from behind the curtain and ask if she would like to speak to me.

"Who are you?" she asks. I introduce myself, saying I want to speak to her about life in the facility. "Are you from the state?" she asks, "because I have a lot to say about this place!"

I explain I am an independent consultant, hired by the facility to educate staff about the ways in which a resident's quality of life can be improved. I tell her I hope she will help me understand what life is like for residents of this facility, giving me information I will use to make my education sessions more specific to this nursing home. She agrees and opens the curtain.

Cindy is sitting on her bed. She is wearing a tan and white bandana on her head. She sports several tattoos and piercings. Some of the tattoos are symbols associated with witchcraft. The letters tattooed on the knuckles of her right hand spell FUCK. She tells me she loves heavy metal music, music which helps her cope, and gestures to the earbuds around her neck.

She presents a tough exterior, uses profanity, and announces "I don't take any crap." After using the word *fuck* three or four times in one sentence, she pauses and chuckles to herself. "Excuse my French," she says, smiling, "I don't mean to offend you." When I tell her it's not a word that's new to me, so I'm neither shocked nor offended, she seems disappointed.

The space around Cindy's bed is cluttered with clothing, snacks, books, bags, and other assorted belongings. Things are piled on top of other things. Things are piled on her bed and on her wheelchair, and still more things are under the bed. I comment on the clutter.

"Nobody helps me here," she says. "I have nowhere to put my stuff. They don't even help me put on these damn (compression) stockings!" She complains her room is too crowded, and that her elderly roommates keep her up at night by calling out. She can't wait to get out of here.

I ask if we can find a place to talk. She responds it is *smoke time*, one of only three scheduled, monitored times each day: 8 a.m., 1 p.m., and 6 p.m. Miss one and wait for the next one, which Cindy – a heavy smoker – does not intend to do.

To follow the staff smoking monitor to the designated outdoor area, Cindy transfers herself from her bed to her wheelchair with ease, attaching the foot pedals independently. She declines my offer to wheel her to our destination, and propels her chair independently without difficulty. When we arrive, we join seven other residents of various ages. All line up to receive a single cigarette and a light from the smoking monitor, and they all want to know who I am.

"She's an advocate," Cindy tells them. "She's going to make some changes around here. She's going to make it better for me and you and the other inmates."

Cindy and I move away from the others at her suggestion. She doesn't want anyone to overhear out conversation, which begins when I ask how she came to live in this facility. Here is her story:

> *I was diagnosed with multiple sclerosis (MS) several years ago. It made my legs weak and I fell several times. I was admitted here for physical therapy following one of those falls. I was discharged back home, but I couldn't make it on my own. I was using heroin and I overdosed and had a stroke. That's is why I'm here for the third time.*
>
> *I know I can be selfish and I've done many things that were painful for my children and other people who care about me. I regret a lot of things I did when I was young. I wish the two kids I lost to foster care and adoption would give me a second chance. I got back in touch with them recently – a son and a daughter. My daughter thinks she might like a relationship with me, but my son does not. His life hasn't been good and he blames me and my selfishness.*
>
> *I know he is angry, and I feel guilty for what I've done. But I'm angry too. I have trouble remembering things and I get frustrated. I lose my temper and I get depressed. That's why I use drugs; they make me feel better. Heroin takes away the pain. When I'm high I don't have to think about anyone or anything.*

Cindy finishes her cigarette as the smoking monitor closes shop. We follow others into the building, as I suggest we find a quiet place to resume our conversation. She agrees to accompany me to a small sitting room where our talk continues in private.

Once seated, I thank her for taking the time to talk with me. I ask her to tell me more about her life here and her plans to return to a home in the community.

During the next hour, she describes many problems with the facility's environment. She is particularly unhappy about the way the staff interacts with her. They give her no privacy and she feels caged, as if she were in prison. "I'm not even allowed to fucking go outside!"

She says staff members don't meet her needs. She says they play favorites, showing fondness for some residents and giving them preferential treatment. Staff members make her wait for help while they provide service to others. As an example, she complains about waiting more than hour for the hot water she uses to make coffee or tea. Since the facility won't allow residents unsupervised access to hot water for safety reasons, she must depend on staff members to provide it and they respond too slowly.

Another complaint: her caregivers are always changing. She never knows who's going to care for her or when they will arrive, a lack of coordination prompting her to refuse care.

She soothes her frustrations by listening to music, which helps her cope. Smoking helps, too. She admits to "talking loudly" to her roommates. "I talk loudly to Edna because she is hard of hearing. I tell her to ring the bell, ring the bell! A lot of times, she doesn't get it." She denies being abusive to her elderly peers. "Hey, I'm no abuser. I respect these old people."

The conversation eventually returns to her plans for discharge. She tells me about her boyfriend. He is looking for apartments and helping her organize the various documents she needs for housing applications. They have also spent time in recent weeks packing her things in anticipation of discharge.

Her housing options are limited, due both to her disability and criminal history. Public housing doesn't accept anyone with a criminal history. Her need for personal care and assistance rules out other properties.

There are several other barriers to overcome, but she is adamant about going home and staying home. She has one grandchild and another on the way. Her plans include spending quality time with her grandchildren, showing herself to them as a better person than she was when she was raising their parents.

When I ask how she will sustain herself this time, she names her boyfriend as the stabilizing factor. For health care, she will rely on Medicaid; for income there are Social Security benefits and food stamps. She expects her housing will be subsidized.

When I ask her if she plans to work, she laughs. She doesn't think about working because she believes her disability makes it impossible. Once I tell her how the Internet now makes it possible for many people with disabilities to work from home, she shows interest in the idea.

The Intervention:

After my conversation with Cindy, I convene a meeting with the interdisciplinary team directly involved in her care: social worker, unit nurse, primary nursing assistant, and activity leader. Cindy's boyfriend accepts an invitation to join us.

The meeting results in a plan which considers Cindy's cognitive needs, as well as her emotional and tangible needs. It addresses her concerns, as well as those of her caregivers, and the following interventions were agreed upon and reflected in it:

1. Cindy will:
   a. Work with the director of social services to continue the discharge planning process;
   b. Request any necessary assistance to access and print her Social Security income statement or her credit report;
   c. Work with her boyfriend to change her mailing address so that her mail is sent to the facility;
   d. Work with her boyfriend and care team members to organize her room and the documents necessary for housing applications and financial planning;
   e. Work with her primary CNA and nurse to develop a care routine that meets the needs of all parties. The routine must include agreement as to the scheduled times for assistance with Activities of Daily Living (ADL), as well as the rules for changes to this schedule by either party;
   f. Work with the facility's nurse practitioner (NP), her community counselor, and her social worker to identify and apply better coping skills when she experiences frustration or anger.

2. The team will:
   a. Provide encouragement and support in organizing Cindy's room and belongings, providing additional storage containers or other options for storing items appropriately;
   b. Provide a dry-erase board in Cindy's room to be updated each shift with the name of her primary CNA and nurse;
   c. Give Cindy a written copy of the ADL schedule once it is cooperatively developed so that it can be jointly reviewed if there is a conflict;
   d. Assist Cindy in using, keeping, and appropriately caring for a thermos of hot water for her beverages. This includes safety education and an evaluation of her ability to comply with the rules for safe and proper use before the intervention is implemented;
   e. Explore all opportunities to help Cindy improve her response to stress, frustration, and anger. The impact of grief and stress on her already compromised situation will be considered and directly addressed through individual counseling. The team will support a plan that includes diversionary activities the resident enjoys, as well as the chance to explore vocational and recreational opportunities that may support her plans for accomplishing and sustaining her discharge.
   f.

The Conclusion:

Like many caregiving teams with which I've worked, this interdisciplinary group had become frustrated with its inability to resolve Cindy's challenging behavior. It had started focusing on the way she expressed her anxiety and frustration, rather than on the underlying clinical and psychosocial circumstances that had an impact on her behavior.

Given her age, diagnoses, physical and cognitive deficits, and her complicated social history, expecting her to be reasonable, control her emotions, and "just get along" was highly unrealistic. In this case, the caregiving team was too close to the situation and too emotionally involved to see past her behavior. In the team's eyes, she had become her behavior.

When this happens, real needs are misinterpreted. Because she has short-term memory issues, she probably doesn't remember what she tells her CNA about her ADL preferences. Since the team was not factoring memory loss into its assessment, it did not initially respond with a practical intervention. By rethinking the issue and by restructuring the care plan to include a written, signed ADL schedule for daily review, it found a way to minimize arguments about it, particularly because the resident now has a copy of it.

Two significant issues were also overlooked by the team: Cindy's heroin addiction history, and the fact that her MS symptoms had escalated and resulted in some cognitive decline.

While her active drug use may have ceased with admission, research indicates that addictive drugs cause changes in the brain that result in cravings and impulsive behavior long afterward. [10]

Cindy's earlier discharges were unsuccessful because only physical accommodations were part of the plan. Little attention was paid to helping her find the external motivation to refrain from self-damaging behavior while living independently. As a result, she relapsed each time, setting off a chain reaction: she lands back in the facility with greater frustration and more negative behavior than with the previous readmission.

The impact of MS on her mood and behavior should have been another critical consideration. As MS progresses – and Cindy's symptoms had intensified since her previous admissions – people can experience a variety of mood disturbances and psychiatric symptoms. Paranoid ideas, irritability, increased libido, and alcohol and substance abuse are all associated with the diagnosis.[11] To

---

10 Bevilacqua, L. and Goldman, D. "Genes and Addiction." National Center for Biotechnology. ncbi.nlm.nih.gov. **https://www.ncbi.nlm.nih.gov/pmc/articles/PMC2715956/**. (Accessed June 23, 2017)

11 Haussleiter, Ida S., Brune, Martin, and Juckel, Georg. "Psychopathology in Multiple Sclerosis." National Center for Biotechnology. ncbi.nlm.nih.gov. **https://www.ncbi.nlm.nih.gov/pmc/articles/PMC3002616/**. (Accessed July 10, 2017)

cope with such symptoms, and to manage the cravings related to her earlier addiction, Cindy needs appropriate therapy. Without appropriate therapeutic intervention and life skills programming to address her coping skills and emotional well-being, her recovery will be superficial.

It is true that psychiatric and addiction counseling services are not readily available to nursing homes located in rural areas, such as this one. The alternative is psychiatric and addiction counseling via teleconferencing, an increasingly popular and practical option in areas where consultant services in some specialties are sparse. Before Cindy is discharged again, her caregiving team will exercise such an option, providing her with the necessary therapy.

The Take-Away

The process described here is assessment and care planning at its best. There was a comprehensive assessment of the person and her circumstances. It was followed by a discussion with the individual in question as to what she needs and wants from the caregiving team. That opened a new dialogue between the resident and the caregivers that was truly person-centered and person-directed.

All caregiving teams should carefully examine how they assess the circumstances leading to admission. Many times, analyzing pre-admission circumstances provides the best clues to the most realistic expectations of resident behavior.

In this case, much of what was described to me as *behavior* turned out to be a typical response for someone with Cindy's profile. By changing its focus to her psychiatric, cognitive, and addiction needs, the team expedites her recovery and gives her the proper preparation to live independently.

It is difficult for any long-term care facility to uphold a standard of care when it doesn't always have the resources for adequate staffing and equipment. In this case, the team lacked the clinical skills or the immediate resources necessary to address psychiatric and addiction issues, and the daily stress of the caregiving environment distorted its perspective.   Overwhelmed, it was difficult for the team to see the solitary tree in the great big forest and objectivity was lost.

Sometimes, it is wise to enlist an objective third party, such as an ombudsman or pastoral counselor, as a moderator during care discussions because it makes it easier to achieve care compromises. Remember, the goal is always a reasonable, person-centered care plan that can be accomplished and sustained, something that is impossible without compromise.

four
Helga

The Individual:

Helga (86) has multiple diagnoses:
   Alzheimer's disease, anxiety, high blood pressure, and Type 2 diabetes.

The Challenging Behavior:

Described by staff as alert but confused with respect to time, place, and situation, Helga often resists care related to Activities of Daily Living (ADL). She sometimes yells or strikes out at the staff. Her husband, who lives in the community, visits her daily for several hours. She does not always recognize him as her husband, and sometimes calls him Daddy.
   Helga has recently begun to cry uncontrollably when he prepares to go home, and she calls after him as he leaves. Staff members say she tries to follow him to the lobby and, when they attempt to redirect her, she can react with anger. Sometimes she strikes out at them. Once he is gone from the building it may be several hours before Helga engages in any activity.

The History:

Described by family as quiet and patient, Helga was never known to raise her voice or be aggressive. Formerly a dedicated elementary school teacher, Helga continued to meet monthly with her colleagues for lunch after she retired. She and her husband traveled extensively and she loves to read. A Roman Catholic of Polish decent, she finds comfort in her faith and identifies with Polish culture and cuisine. She always wears a rosary.

The Current Situation:

Before admission, Helga's husband was caring for her at home with the help of a home health care worker. In the early stages of her illness, she might forget where she'd left something, or she might put dishes away in the wrong place. As her illness progressed, her memory loss worsened and, like many people with Alzheimer's disease or dementia, she began "Sundowning."[12]

The term Sundowning describes confusion occurring in late afternoon and spanning into night. It isn't a disease, but a group of symptoms categorized by the time of day in which they emerge. It can manifest in anxiety or aggression, and can lead to pacing or wandering.

In the months before moving to the nursing home, Helga had begun wandering at night. Once, she left the house while her husband was sleeping. He awoke to find her gone, called the police, and reported her missing. She was found several hours later, walking in the parking lot of the nearby grocery store, and the police brought her home.

As much as it troubled them, the incident forced the family to consider other living options. This escalation of her symptoms, along with her husband's failing health, made them realize that living at home was no longer safe for Helga. As reluctant as he was to accept long-term care as the inevitable option, her husband was diligent in researching the best match for Helga's circumstances. With regret, and great guilt, he admitted her to the nursing home.

---

12 Graff-Radford, M.D., Jonathan. "Sundowning: Late-day Confusion." Mayo Clinic. Mayoclinic.org.

http://www.mayoclinic.org/diseases-conditions/alzheimers-disease/expert-answers/sundowning/faq-20058511. (Accessed June 23, 2017)

The Assessment:

I interviewed Helga using several props to stimulate her memory. In the mid to late stages of dementia, aphasia and other communication deficits are sometimes present. Aphasia may cause difficulties in speaking, listening, reading, and writing, but does not affect intelligence; likewise, certain dementias inhibit language but not necessarily cohesive thought. Props such as flash cards of everyday items, or photographs of people and places someone has known, can help bring words forward.

It is also a good idea to insert information the person provides into the successive interview questions. It not only extends the exchange, but also makes the conversation feel increasingly familiar to him or her. Such familiarity generally makes it easier for the individual to engage.

For example, I ask Helga to tell me her husband's name. She can't remember it. I say it's not important and turn our attention to her family photographs. As we look at pictures taken when she was much younger, she mentions Michael. "Is Michael your husband?" I ask. "No," she says, "he is my brother." Now that I know who Michael is, I can use his name to move the conversation forward.

In another photograph, she points to herself and a young boy. "Who is that?" I ask. "That's Thomas, my cousin," she replies. Now I have two names to use to help me help her make connections that may bring more of her memory forward.

Looking at a picture of several men posing on a dock with fish they caught, I ask if Michael is in the picture. She points to Michael. "Is Thomas in the picture, too?" I ask. "Yes," she says and points him out. When I ask about two other men in the photo, she identifies one as John and the other as Bobby, pointing to them as she recognizes them. "Is John your husband?" I ask. "No." "Is Bobby your husband?" "Yes."

The entire conversation takes approximately fifteen minutes. It is long enough to get her memory working and give it ample time to catch up to the conversation. It is always encouraging for me when so much information is revealed by engaging someone for such a short time.

After the interview, I spent additional time observing Helga's behavior in the general environment. She did not seek out social opportunities, but did mingle with others if prompted by the staff. In the hours before her husband arrived she wandered the hallways looking for him. She asked others if they had seen him. Staff members could engage her in conversation, but were unable to redirect her with board games, dolls, or similar items.

Next, I met with Helga's family: her husband, son, and daughter-in-law. We discussed her earlier life and the ways in which her dementia affected each of them. The information they provided formed the history documented in the first part of this chapter and became the foundation for a person-centered approach to Helga's needs.

The Intervention:

Using the information discovered in Helga's assessment interview, along with insight provided by her family, Helga's caregivers have five ways to intervene:

Socialization: because Helga is willing to interact with others if prompted, the staff will identify other teachers among the residents and organize a small social group. The group will meet in a quiet area away from excessive activity, and members will be encouraged to share memories common to them as teachers. Pictures of classroom activities, as well as actual tools teachers use, are props that can be used to stimulate memory and discussion.

Engagement: Since one of the facility's housekeepers reported that Helga sometimes reads to her, staff will encourage Helga to read aloud more often. It may be possible to have her read to a small group of other residents in a quiet area, or suggest she read to her husband when he visits. If a novel or poem she once loved can be identified, she can be encouraged to read it aloud. Plan this activity in the morning to avoid the chance of afternoon Sundowning. Offer a player with headphones so Helga can listen to an audio book in her room or in a quiet section of the common area.

Heritage: Since Helga still identifies with her Polish ethnic heritage and culture, the staff should share with her photographs, music, artifacts, or videos of the country and its people in a private, quiet setting. If possible, consider a hands-on activity involving ethnic food preparation such as pierogi. Both techniques are likely to stimulate fond memories, which can lead to calmer and more cooperative interactions.

Faith: While Helga routinely attends religious services, she may find additional comfort in an individualized faith experience. Since she always wears a rosary, she may find it soothing if someone on staff says a portion of the rosary with her. Likewise, having a staff member sit quietly with her in the chapel during late afternoon may help diminish the anxiety that can accompany Sundowning.

Recollection: The staff should attempt to elicit memories that may sometimes prompt Helga to recognize and identify with her husband as he is today. The family should be asked to participate in creating photo boards that include:

- A chronological display of Helga and her husband at various stages of their relationship, starting with the earliest photos and progressing to the present. This may eliminate her inclination to confuse her husband with her father. A similar display involving Helga's son should also be created.
- A thematic display of travels taken with the family
- photographs of the home she shared with her family and events that took place there Helga's husband should be asked to recount stories from their travels, particularly funny ones, when he visits. Those stories should be repeated by caregivers to encourage Helga to see them as people who really "know" her. Staff should also help Helga journal, or record her own memories, as another excellent one-on-one activity that may provide comfort and calming.

It may also be helpful to develop a memory box. The box should contain Helga's personal photographs and keepsakes. When she is in distress, staff members can encourage her to review the items in the box. She may be comforted by them. If the box is created, it must be kept intact and stored in a common location. There must be easy access to it either by Helga herself, or by staff members who are providing it to her.

Finally, identifying favorite songs and making such music available to her is another way to allow recollection to prevent the onset of negative thoughts or feelings.

All the activities described above are more appropriate for someone at Helga's stage of dementia than the dolls or board games the staff typically offers. Dolls, building blocks and games are better utilized when people enter the childlike states typical of late stage dementia. Before that, residents are more likely to see such as items as what they are: toys. Toys are for children, not for them.

In addition to these formal interventions, there are some simple adjustments family and staff can make that will minimize Helga's distress. Her husband can refrain from saying goodbye as he is leaving because it triggers crying and agitation. By quietly retreating without an overt exit signal he can diminish such emotionally-charged reactions.

If Helga enjoys listening to music and can use headphones, it is another way to soothe and distract her from her husband's exit. He might offer the headphones to her and start the music so that she is engaged in a pleasurable activity as he leaves. Depending on her short-term recall, it's possible she may not remember he has come and gone.

Similarly, staff shift changes should be accomplished quietly – no saying goodbye to coworkers or calling out "see you tomorrow." Not having to overhear such comments can help eliminate Helga's feeling of being left behind and the resulting anguish.

The Conclusion:

Helga was initially described to me in a generic way: a woman who cries uncontrollably and tries to elope from the unit. Yet by asking questions about her crying, and gathering details about how and when it happens, we put together the triggers: Sundowning, her husband's departure, and late day fatigue. Identifying the triggers made the behavior more comprehensible and more amenable to intervention.

Taking the next step, learning Helga's customary routines in terms of home, work, faith, and socialization, allowed a fuller picture of the woman to emerge: who she was and how she lived her life before she had a dementia diagnosis. By looking at that holistic image we found our clues to the care plan that would improve her quality of life.

Of the many potential interventions suggested for Helga, some worked well and others were unsuccessful. She cried less if her husband left without saying goodbye; the photo displays helped her distinguish her husband from her father, and she was better able to recognize her son if she saw a picture of him that included her and her husband.

She continued reading aloud to the housekeeper who cleans her room every morning. However, she was only willing to read to others if it were a small group and she was asked to do it in a small lounge at the end of the hallway. She had fleeting interest in looking at books or other teaching tools, and engaged in only brief conversation about teaching when prompted. After a time, her language skills deteriorated and she was unable to successfully communicate with others.

By working through the challenges presented by a single individual, the care team learned how to develop more effective interventions, how important it is to tailor them to individual ability, and that it is critical to identify more than one type of remedy. No single remedy works for everyone and none of them work forever. Interventions must be modified as the dementia progresses, so that they are fluid and keep pace with an individual's unique needs.

The Take-Away

Many of the behaviors that strike us as odd or unusual are often common-place reactions to an individual's perception of his or her experience. It becomes a problem when caregivers don't understand the individual's perception. Too often, professional caregivers overlook the importance of a holistic assessment.

In caring for someone with dementia, a mental disorder, or a brain injury, the assessment process must extend to life events, relationships, personality and the customary behavior of the individual. Otherwise, there is no hope of understanding why people do what they do. They become one-dimensional. They become the behavior.

five
John

The Individual:

John (67) has a paranoid schizophrenia diagnosis. He shows symptoms of Tardive Dyskinesia (TD), a movement disorder associated with prolonged use of antipsychotic medication. Its symptoms are primarily characterized by random movements of different muscles and the tongue, lips, or jaw. In John's case, it manifests as uncontrolled leg movement.[13]

The Challenging Behavior:

After John contracted a virus that resulted in a respiratory infection and a skin rash, he became convinced that it was the building's electricity, not the virus, that caused his illness. He informed the charge nurse that it was the new light bulbs installed in the hallway adjacent to his room that were sickening him and, consequently, he was now unable to leave his room. He insisted that meals be delivered to him in his room, and he stopped attending any activity outside of his room. His socialization with others was dramatically diminished.

Both the resident social worker and a psychologist engaged him, challenging his conclusions. When they explained that the virus

---

13 National Alliance on Mental Illness. "Tardive Dyskinesia." nami.org. **https://www.nami.org/Learn-More/Mental-Health-Conditions/Related-Conditions/Tardive-Dyskinesia**. (Accessed June 23, 2017)

that caused his illness had spread throughout the facility and caused problems for others, John became defensive. He became angry and shouted at them.

The History

John is of German heritage and lived in Frankfurt, Germany as a young man. He was a tailor's assistant as he worked his way through school. He studied economics, and his dream was to own a clothing factory.

In his junior year of school, he began experiencing symptoms of schizophrenia. He suffered delusions and thought other students were stealing his ideas. He had auditory hallucinations in which he believed he heard a friend telling him which students were stealing from him. Because the auditory "friend" told him the ideas were stolen telepathically he started always wearing a cap. He believed the cap prevented anyone from accessing the ideas in his brain.

Eventually his symptoms escalated to a psychotic episode that resulted in brief hospitalization. At the hospital, he was medicated for schizophrenia and his symptoms lessened. For the next several years the medication was a stabilizing influence, allowing him to finish school and live a relatively normal life. His symptoms were not as intense, though he still experienced some sense of discomfort he later describes as "I just didn't feel right."

After he was graduated from school he applied for and was awarded an apprenticeship at a clothing manufacturing company in Pennsylvania. He emigrated to the United States and, feeling better, stopped his medication. He was successful in his life and his work for about four years before intensified symptoms of schizophrenia disrupted him.

Like many people who have schizophrenia, John had the mistaken impression that the medication he took in Germany had cured him. He stopped using it because he felt so much better. He didn't understand that it was the medication itself that was responsible for his improvement; without it, he would experience the same or worse difficulties as before.

It was the beginning of a debilitating cycle: hospitalization, medication, stabilization, and release; improvement, stopped medication, and relapse. In the end, he was committed to the state's psychiatric hospital, assessed as lacking the capacity to care for his own health and well-being.

John lived at the hospital for 23 years, until The Community Mental Health Act of 1963 prompted wide release of institutionalized individuals into less restrictive environments. He was placed in the nursing home, as were many of the people he had been friendly with at the state hospital.

The Current Situation

John is friendly with the staff and remains friends with other residents who had lived along with him at the state hospital. Many of these people look to John as a leader because he went to college and is bilingual. In the years he has lived in the nursing home there have been no incidents of aggressive behavior or unexplained agitation. His insistence that the building's electricity is making him sick is the first time John has presented the staff with an unworkable challenge.

The Assessment:

When I interview John, I find him to be intelligent and well-spoken. He expresses himself clearly, and gives what sounds to be a very rational, detailed explanation of how the electricity gets inside his body through the top of his head. He likens this problem to his early college days when others were stealing his ideas by plucking them from the top of his head.

I ask him why the electricity that powers the lights and the clock in his room is not making him sick. He looks at me, leans in, and speaking in a whisper says, "That electricity was given to Benjamin Franklin by God, so it will not harm me."

The Intervention:

Since John is comfortable with the electricity in his room, I ask if I may bring a record player into his room. He enjoys German opera and has not had the opportunity to listen to music since his self-imposed isolation began.

He is eager to hear the music and agrees to allow me to use the Benjamin Franklin electricity to power the record player. We enjoy several mornings of music, but John still declines invitations to attend music activities outside of his room.

Trying to minimize his isolation, I ask if we can invite several of his friends to his room to listen to the music together. He agrees, and he and I and other residents enjoy several more days of musical programming in his room.

Two months into this effort to address John's fear of the electricity, a free concert is scheduled for a Sunday afternoon in a local park. Many are interested in going, so arrangements are made to take a group to the concert. I share the information with John, encouraging him to join the group because I think he would really enjoy the music.

John considers the suggestion for a moment, but declines. He is still fearful of the electricity in the hallway. He reasons there is no way he can travel from his room to the exit of the building without being exposed to the harmful hallway electricity and he does not want to get sick again.

Disappointed that the last several weeks of work with John has not diminished his fear, I am determined to discover another solution. My fear is that the longer he isolates himself, the more his condition will decline. I want him to return to the mainstream of facility life and enjoy himself. How can I help him protect himself from his belief that the dangerous electricity will enter his body?

I think about umbrellas ... that they protect you from the elements. I discover a new type of umbrella, one that is fashioned from clear plastic and extends over the body so that it protects it all the way to the knees. I buy one for John and offer it to him. I let him know that I believe this umbrella will protect him from the dangerous electricity if he wears it when he leaves his room.

John is skeptical, not so much of the umbrella but of me. He smiles and asks if I am joking. I deny any attempt at humor and emphasize that I have settled on this remedy after researching many others. I tell him I have confidence in this solution and that I really hope it will work. I want him to come with us to the concert and enjoy the music. I suggest we take the umbrella for a test run and he agrees.

With the umbrella engaged, we leave his room and walk down the hall toward the front entrance. As we are about to exit outside, I ask him how he is feeling. "Is the umbrella protecting you, John? Do you feel any ill effects from the electricity?" He does not. He smiles, walks through the front door and into the sunshine for the first time in months.

In the weeks that followed, John used the umbrella to attend many programs in the facility and out in the community. He had such a good time at an Oktoberfest celebration that he forgot to use his umbrella when we returned to the facility.

The next day, I asked John how he was feeling. "Good," was the answer and he said again how much he enjoyed the concert. "Do you realize you didn't wear the umbrella when we returned from the concert?" I asked. "I didn't?" he said. "No, John, and you're fine today, aren't you?"

We then had a conversation about the fact that he suffered no adverse effects from the electricity even though many hours had passed since he walked through the hallway without the umbrella. I suggested we step out into the hallway to see if there would be any problem. He agreed and there was none.

He never used the umbrella again, remained healthy, and continued to live his full and happy life when I last saw him.

The Conclusion:

The first step in resolving any challenging behavior is to develop a positive, trusting relationship with the individual. In this case, the many mornings I spent with John listening to music and enjoying it together formed a bond. He had trust in me and, as a result, was trustful of the idea I presented.

In cases where schizophrenia is present, it can be helpful to refrain from either validating or denying the underlying reason for the behavior. Instead, it can be more successful to focus on a solution that addresses the issue: in John's case, it was adequate protection from what he perceived as a threat to his well-being.

I had no idea if the umbrella would work, but I knew that umbrellas offered protection from the elements. I knew, too, that John was primarily concerned about the effect on his brain, making me think that in covering his head he would feel safe. That's one key to successful interventions: try new, even offbeat ideas, and don't be deterred by the potential for defeat.

The Take-Away

When working with someone diagnosed with a mental disorder, recognize that finding the correct, personalized intervention will take time. There is no blueprint to a solution that works for all people with the same diagnosis. Both the assessment and the approach you plan must accommodate and be tailored to the individual's unique needs.

As a caregiver, try not to be limited by your perception of reality. Try meeting individuals where they are, listening to their concerns and attempting to alleviate them.

In other words, experiment and use your personal creativity to help you address some of the more challenging behavioral health issues.

six

Bonnie Mae

The Individual

Bonnie Mae (86) has an Alzheimer's diagnosis. She is in the middle to late stages of dementia, though her language skills are intact. She can make herself understood and she can respond to questions. While she occasionally forgets or struggles with words, most of her conversation is clear. She does not remember her husband's name or recognize her adult children when they visit.

The Challenging Behavior

Bonnie Mae does not exist in the present. Oriented instead in various phases of her earlier life, she becomes angry and agitated when staff members contradict the details she shares with them. Told, for example, that her children are adults now and they no longer depend on her to make their lunches or pick them up from school, Bonnie Mae lashes out. She calls her caregivers liars, accusing them of keeping her a prisoner and away from the children who need her. Her frustrations often escalate to the point that she attempts to "escape" the facility.

The History

Bonnie Mae became a resident seven months ago. She had been living in the community in a home she shared with her husband. He was her primary caregiver. Once he passed away, Bonnie Mae was admitted to the nursing home.

When she was first admitted, Bonnie Mae behaved as if she was still as a young married woman and frequently expressed concerns about the well-being of her young children. Recently she has regressed to an earlier stage of her life and has no memory of her marriage or her children. She doesn't recall living in the local community and tells the staff she arrived here from Alabama, though she has not lived there since she was a girl.

The Current Situation

While Bonnie Mae once participated in activity programs, especially those focused on music or word games, she can no longer tolerate a group setting. Large numbers of people and excessive noise and activity disturb her. She now tells others to be quiet and lays individual claim to an activity table. If other residents attempt to sit at her table, she shoos them away saying she's waiting for her friends to arrive. The others are offended by her commands to be quiet and her attempts to relocate them. Arguments inevitably follow.

Lately, Bonnie Mae also spends part of the day stacking dirty dishes at the nurses' station, a behavior the staff would like to end. The objective is to find ways to engage Bonnie Mae so that she is less disruptive and there are fewer reasons for her to become agitated by others or by the general environment.

The Assessment:

On the afternoon I am asked to evaluate her, I find Bonnie Mae in the dining room. Lunch for her unit is over and her meal has ended.

She busy removing dirty plates from the lunch truck, dirty plates that were being readied to return to the kitchen. Instead, Bonnie Mae is taking the dishes to the nurses' station and stacking them on the counter there. She is loudly complaining about the residents, offended by what "pigs" they are and how much food they waste.

A CNA approaches and tries to take the dishes from her, explaining the dishes must go back on the truck so that they can return to the kitchen where they will be washed. Bonnie Mae resists her, insisting that removing the dishes is her job. A tug-of-war ensues, dishes crash to the floor, and Bonnie Mae begins yelling at the CNA.

I motion for the CNA to move away and leave Bonnie Mae to her task. I observe for a few more minutes, listening as she continues to complain about her "job" and the person who just now tried to keep her from earning a living.

As I approach her I say: "Excuse me, is lunch over?" She looks at me as if she's trying to decide if she knows me, and then replies, "Yes, all done. Uh huh!" She turns back to her task and continues talking about how much she dislikes this "job."

"How did you get this job?" I ask. When she answers that her mother got the job for her, I follow up with: "Oh, I see. May I ask how old you are?" "I'm sixteen," she replies, "and I'll be seventeen in October."

I ask her why she continues to do this job if she doesn't like it. She says times are tough and her family needs the money. It's the reason she had to leave high school early. She dreams of getting married and starting a family, but she must work until that happens.

The Intervention:

This is an opportunity to practice validation: rather than reason with someone who has lost the ability to reason, it's better to listen closely to what the person is saying, try to understand the thinking, and find a way to enter the conversation on his or her terms. It's the approach widely recommended by dementia care experts.

Applying it in Bonnie Mae's situation, I continue to talk with her while she finishes her "job" of cleaning up. I remind her that most people must work their entire adult lives, even after they marry and start families. Since she is so young, it may mean that she will work for fifty years or more. "If I were you," I tell her, "I wouldn't keep a job I didn't like. I'd quit and find a better job." I spend the next few minutes encouraging her to do just that.

"No, no," she says, "my mother would be angry. We need the money."

With that, I tell her that a better job may pay more money and I recount my own early experience in a job I disliked. After leaving it for a job I liked much better, I was not only happier, I was better paid. I enjoyed going to work once I had the right job for me.

"Bonnie Mae," I ask, "what type of job would you like to have?" She can't answer that question, but she is sure this is not the job for her. After another ten minutes of conversation and encouragement, she says yes! She is going to quit her job! She puts the dishes down and wipes her hands. "I'm going to tell my mama I'm done with this nonsense. I quit!" And, looking directly into my eyes, she quietly says, "Thank you."

The Conclusion:

It can be difficult for professional caregivers to know when to attempt to reason with a resident and when to simply listen and validate his or her thoughts. In situations where dementia is a contributing factor, knowing when to choose validation can mean the difference between a relatively simple and calm redirection or an anxious confrontation. It is so often recommended by dementia care experts because they know it is pointless to try to impose reality on people who live within their personal, fragmented memory.[14]

In Bonnie Mae's case, knowing she could recall her life only until she was 16 had me adjust my conversation accordingly. I talked with her the way I would with any teenager. Had she said she was 35, our conversation would have taken a more mature direction. The intervention was successful because I met Bonnie Mae where she was in that moment.

---

14 Feil, Naomi. "What is Validation?" Validation Training Institute, Inc. vfvalidation.org. **https://vfvalidation.org/what-is-validation/**. (Accessed March 18, 2017)

The Take-Away

When working with people who have a dementia diagnosis, it is important to know both the type of dementia they have and the impact it is having on the individual's thinking and functionality. Equally important, however, it to understand the individual on a personal level. Who was he before the dementia took hold? How did she live her life before the diagnosis? This information is critical to knowing how to sustain a quality of life the individual can no longer sustain alone.

With comprehensive, holistic assessment, there is the foundation for person-centered care that allows for as fulfilling a life as possible for as long as possible.

seven

Young Adult Workshop

The Individuals:

A group of six young adults, ranging in age 37 - 56, live in a nursing home that typically serves the frail elderly. They are there because they have disabilities that make them incapable of living independently in the community, and they are part of a larger shift in nursing home populations.

Not only are these residents younger and with fewer age-related physical issues than the elders, they have more complex behavioral and psychosocial concerns. They are also less likely to adjust to institutional living than their aging counterparts.

Three of the six have a bipolar depression diagnosis, and of these one is also affected by anxiety. Two others have a traumatic brain injury: one due to an automobile accident while driving under the influence; the other due to longstanding drug abuse. The sixth member of the group has a schizophrenia diagnosis, has delusions, and was self-medicating with drugs and alcohol before admission.

The Challenging Behavior:

As a group, these residents make the environment uncomfortable for their elderly neighbors. They can be found yelling, using profanity, playing loud music, or watching television late at night at a volume that disturbs others. In general, their elderly peers are terrorized by them. The clinical team has addressed the behavior individually and collectively on many occasions, without success.

To date, the primary incentive for improved behavior is a negative one: behave better or face discharge. For the group members, this is a disincentive: since none of them asked to be admitted to the facility and all have repeatedly expressed a desire to leave it, the idea that disruptive behavior may result in discharge is welcome. It prompts the group to find even more creative ways to generate a chaotic environment.

The History:

Each member of the group has a similar troubling story. In all cases, family support was lacking. All acknowledge that their lifestyles and behaviors put tremendous stress on their relationships with family and friends, and they each feel that they have "burned those bridges."

Two of the people diagnosed with bipolar depression had attempted suicide, one more than once, and both had been homeless.

The individual beset with both bipolar depression and anxiety described a long history of doctors, medications, and unsuccessful attempts to stop using drugs. During manic episodes, this woman was often a risk taker, behaving promiscuously and stealing money to pay for drugs.

The remaining three group members cited abusive or alcoholic parents, poor school and social histories, and some criminal activities as events that led to their current situations. All had turned to traditional medicine for help, but with no success.

The Current Situation:

Part of the caregivers' strategy for diffusing the group's difficult behavior was to allow the members to socialize on the facility's outdoor patio. It allowed them to "get away from the old people," as the group categorized it, and it gave the staff a respite from providing constant correction.

Now that it is winter, with snow on the ground and increasingly cold temperatures, the patio is closed and unavailable to the group.

Forced to remain inside, without the ability to avoid elderly neighbors, the group begins to show signs of cabin fever. Cabin fever causes extreme irritability and restlessness, and the condition is thought to be brought about by living in isolation or in a confined indoor area for a prolonged time.[15]

The Assessment:

I arrange to interview the residents both individually and as a group. It was in the individual interviews that I learned each person's history; in the group interview I focused on its views of its current situation.

Asked about their daily routines in the facility, all complained of boredom, of not having anything to do, and of feeling as though the days are long and pointless. Each wanted something more interesting and productive than the typical Bingo games or sing-a-longs.

When I asked if they would be interested in real work and real earning power, the answer was an enthusiastic, unanimous, "Yes!" Were they willing to commit to a project that would bring them both productivity and income, and would require daily participation in a workshop? Again, a resounding, "Yes!" It's settled. The intervention will be an Activity Workshop.

The Intervention:

Activity Workshops are therapeutic in that they are designed to promote self-esteem and improved mood and behavior through accomplishment and reward. They can take many forms, but are always similar in one important way: they promote dignity and self-actualization among the participants.

In establishing a workshop at this facility, it was decided that it would be an autonomous organization. Residents who participated were to be responsible for workshop environment maintenance, ensuring that it is clean, comfortable, and safe.

---

15 https://www.merriam-webster.com/dictionary/cabin%20fever

The inventory would be maintained by the participants, and they would develop the rules by which everyone was expected to abide.

To ensure the workshop's success, the facility developed a policy and procedure statement. Among the items it defined were the expected therapeutic benefits and incremental improvements in behavior; the standards by which group social behavior was to be evaluated; and the penalties for violating policy and procedure. The statement formed the basis of a contract, one signed by all group members and the staff. Group members each received a copy of the contract and the document was appended to the plan of care.

In this case, the workshop was supported by a Token Economy System[16] Each participant received a daily stipend for productivity. The facility made an initial investment of $100, expecting the workshop to sustain itself financially through the sale of items created by its participants. Half the sale profits were to go into the Token account; the other half to be spent to replenish inventory.

Since a successful workshop must be designed to not only improve group behavior, but to benefit everyone individually, it was important that the preparation for this group's workshop include interviews focused on understanding each member's perceptions: how does each one think and feel about where life has led them? I will not recount all six interviews, but use two as examples.

Consider Horatio (37) who has a traumatic brain injury. He was high on alcohol, as well as the drugs Ecstasy and marijuana, when he was injured in a motor vehicle accident.

Horatio tells me his young life was unsupervised and difficult. His mother was a single parent who worked two jobs and was rarely home. In the age before cell phones, there were times when he and his mother did not see or talk to each other for a couple of days. Food and other necessities were often in short supply, and no one cared if he

---

16 A Token Economy System is a method used for behavioral change that utilizes principles of positive reinforcement. Behavioral Health Works. "How to Use a Token Economy System." bhwcares.com. **http://bhwcares.com/token-economy/**. (Accessed August 5, 2017)

went to school. As he got older, he started socializing with the wrong people. He left school in his freshman year. In a life rife with negative behavior, he turned to drugs as an escape. When he is high, he feels invincible. He says Ecstasy makes him feel strong, powerful, "like I can take out a guy three times my size!"

When I ask him if there is anything about his life to date of which he is genuinely proud, he first describes criminal behavior: fights he won and two convenience store robberies in which he netted a lot of money. "Are those your proudest moments?" I pressed. "Are they the things you want people to remember about you?"

"I've done other stuff," he says. "I used to play basketball in junior high school and I was pretty good." He paused, enjoying the memory, and continued, "I used to like art class, too. Making stuff was cool. One year, I learned how to make jewelry and I made some earrings for this girl I liked. Other girls wanted earrings too, so I started making and selling them."

Asked if he had ever considered making jewelry for a living he looks at me as if to say, "Are you kidding?" He waves his hand and shakes his head no. "Nah, I stopped doing it because some people started saying I was gay. I got into a couple of fights about that, believe me. I showed 'em I ain't no pussy."

In the several conversations that follow, it's clear Horatio hates the life he lives now, and hates confinement in the nursing home. He blames his mother, his school, his neighborhood, and his friends for the way his life turned out. In other words, he blames everyone but himself. There will eventually be a plan of care that helps him more realistically analyze his choices and how they have influenced the current chain of events, but for now I want to focus on the best use of his time in the activity workshop.

Revisiting his comments about making and selling his jewelry in school, I suggest he might make and sell jewelry in the workshop. He's interested in that idea, so I provide him with a few supply catalogs. We order the items he requests and set up a work schedule. Later, we develop pricing and a plan for putting the tokens he earns to good use.

Or, consider Robert. Of the six group members, he is the most disabled when it comes to focus and the ability to sustain productivity. He has a schizophrenia diagnosis, accompanied by paranoia and delusions. He had a long history of hospitalizations, various unsuccessful medication trials, and a deteriorating social circumstance that eventually led to homelessness. Once homeless, he couldn't access the clinical care he needed.

His schizophrenia is currently well-managed. He is following his medication regimen and keeping appointments with his psychologist. His physical health has left him non-ambulatory, dependent on a wheelchair, and in need of skilled care for a foot wound. His loss of independence results in behavior that is sometimes challenging and often prompted by frustration or pain. Even so, he has not initiated any physical altercations.

Like many people with his diagnosis, Robert is very intelligent. Prior to onset at 22, he was a good student and led a relatively normal life. His childhood was unremarkable and he described family events and vacations that were happy and memorable. His relationships with his parents and his brother were once good, but both deteriorated as he sank deeper into his illness.

Asked about his proudest achievements, he mentions his writing. He writes both poems and short stories, and poems are his preference. He likes to write poems about life and love.

Following several conversations about workshop participation, he says he wants to write poems people can purchase as birthday or holiday gifts. The poems can include personal references and he will stencil them onto posters. This unique artistic gift was to become one of the most sought-after birthday presents in the facility, and prompted Robert to expand the idea.

Activity staff helped him discover how he could use the computer to create notecards featuring his poems. He sold them in packages of six, fastened together with decorative bows created by a fellow workshop participant. Their collaboration encouraged others to experiment with shared projects and contributed to the eventual expansion of the workshop program.

The Conclusion:

For each of the original six, the workshop experience helped them lead a more normal and satisfying existence. They now had the opportunity to be productive and to explore their creativity in ways they might not have considered otherwise.

While there were times when each of them might express dissatisfaction, or have a change in mood prompting a pre-workshop type of behavior, the group's opportunity to creatively express itself generated an overall sense of self-esteem and self confidence that kept disruption to a minimum.

In fact, even more positive social group behavior emerged. Participants opted in the first year to bank some tokens and use them to have lunch together at a local restaurant. The collegial atmosphere in which these friendships developed, and the ongoing camaraderie and collective focus necessary to sustain the workshop, helped each member find a quality of life. Life was worth living once more.

The Take-Away:

Once a social group forms, modifying its behavior requires both an understanding of each group member as well as the group dynamics. In this case, the spontaneously formed group was founded on negative behavior and thrived on constant complaints, verbal abuse of elderly peers, and developing new ways to refuse care and challenge and frustrate the staff. As a collective problem, it demanded to be addressed in a collective fashion.

The first step was identifying a common positive goal: be productive and make money. The next step was learning what it would take for each member of the group to embrace the goal – what was it about individual history and perception that would lead to interest and enthusiasm? If even one member lacked sufficient commitment to success, the group would fail. Because the concept was developed in a holistic manner consistent with person-centered care, the group not only abandoned its negative behavior, it blossomed into that had found a source of joy.

As changes in the long-term care census continue, all therapeutic activity programs must be fluid and adaptable to the residents' needs. The workshop was this facility's first attempt to rethink meaningful activity for an increasingly diverse population. It is an excellent example of how important it is that caregivers recognize the roles of productivity and socialization in personal satisfaction and quality of life.

eight

Putting Thought into Action: Steps to Take Toward Person-Centered Care

After reading the case histories included here, my guess is that you are already thinking of ways that holistic assessment may improve the caregiving situation in the long-term care facility where you work. If you want to put those thoughts into action, follow my lead: when asked to evaluate people with agitated or aggressive behavior, do your best to learn as much as you can about them. Find out who the resident was before illness set in, who the resident is now, and what is necessary for the resident to thrive in the current circumstances. Communication or cognitive deficits can make it challenging, but here are the steps to take to form an insightful personal profile that will guide the care plan.

Assign the Assessment Interview to the Primary CNA

If, as the facility's resident social worker you typically complete the initial assessment profile, consider a change in procedure. Suggest the primary CNA begin the assessment process so there in no delay in communicating lifestyle, occupation and family history to the person who needs it most – the person who has day-to-day interaction with the resident in providing intimate care.

On the other hand, if you are the primary CNA, ask the team to assign this role to you. Express confidence that, by welcoming the resident and asking the questions that lead to person-centered care, there will be less disruption over the long-term. Point out that this approach fosters trust, and that trust is the key to resident cooperation in his or her care. After all, who better to welcome a new resident and offer help in adjusting to the new environment than the person who is shortly about to see the resident naked?

Expand the Assessment Questionnaire

Consider adding the following questions, questions not typically found in admission assessment documents, to the assessment interview:

- *What are the known or potential triggers to behavior?* For example, what are the phobias, delusions, or environmental issues such as temperature or noise levels that have an impact on behavior? Likewise, are there personal preferences a resident is no longer able to express verbally that result in disruption when the preferences are denied? An example is the woman who prefers dresses to slacks but, unable to express this verbally, disrobes if forced to wear slacks.
- *What was the pre-illness personality?* If you discover, for example, that a resident has always had a strong personality, accustomed to taking charge and giving orders, it's to be expected that he will continue to exhibit this type of behavior. Once the caregiving team accepts that this is typical for the resident, and not agitated or aggressive behavior, it is better able to find ways to minimize the disruptions the behavior may cause.
- *What is the resident's social and occupational history?* Ask questions that lead to an understanding of the resident's social style. Is he outgoing? Is she an introvert? What type of work did the resident once do? How does the resident feel about status, control, personal reputation, or "keeping up with the Joneses?" Understanding how people perceived themselves in society, both socially and occupationally, can shed some light on behavior the team will be required to address.
- *What are the family dynamics that may have an impact on the resident's interaction with others?* In the case of a memory-impaired resident, a caregiver may bear a resemblance to someone in

the resident's past. The resemblance may trigger a negative response, particularly if the prior relationship was unhealthy. Families do not easily divulge such personal information. To elicit it, start by explaining the need to know to the family and the ways in which the information will be used to comfort the resident.

- *What are the resident's preferences and routines?* While much of this information is reflected in the social history and comprehensive assessment document, knowing the resident's favorite color, song, or pastime can lead to person-centered, diversionary interventions. Toward this goal, ask families to provide photographs, audio/video tapes, or other familiar items that can become part of diversionary activity.

- *What are the traumas the person may have experienced, and how have they influenced mood or behavior?* The federal government will require all long-term care facilities to evaluate residents for post-traumatic stress disorder (PTSD) beginning in 2019. However, as explained in Chapter 2 of this book, PTSD associated with military service or combat experience is only one type of trauma. Many life events may be traumatic. Being robbed, having a terrible motor vehicle accident, suffering a miscarriage or domestic violence, being homeless, or being bullied as a child are all potentially traumatic events. Giving up all the accomplishments and status of a prior life to move into a nursing home should be considered a traumatic event.

The following additional questions are suggested to promote understanding of an individual's personality traits, as well as the lifetime rituals and routines that influence mood and behavior.

1. *How is anger expressed?* Different people express anger, stress or frustration differently. Some yell, some practice the silent treatment, and some slam things such as doors or drawers. Still others display physical aggression, which may be randomly directed. How does this resident exhibit extreme emotion?

2. ***How are large groups of people tolerated?*** In the community, people generally find themselves in groups within several limited situations: work, school, church, a club, a party, or a special event. Most of us spend the bulk of our personal time either alone or with a limited number of family or friends. Consequently, how someone tolerates being in a group every day for extended periods of time is a caregiving item of interest.
3. ***What is soothing or calming during episodes of extreme emotion?*** Smoking a cigarette or a joint, taking a drink, shopping, working out, bathing, sleeping, overeating or simply going for a long drive are among the many ways people release the adrenalin that stems from extreme emotion. What is this resident's customary approach?
4. ***What would be the activity of choice were no obstacles in its path?*** If the resident could do anything that came to mind, what would it be? The answer to this question provides some insight into individual priorities and values and may reveal other information that results in a more robust personality profile. The more robust the profile, the better the chances of developing a blueprint for a person-centered plan of care.

Get the Timing Right

Give careful thought to the timing of the assessment interview, and consider it a two-part process. Start with a session focused on the information necessary for a baseline care plan. The questions should be related to what the caregiving team needs to ensure that the resident's primary needs are met. Allow at least 24 – 48 hours to go by before scheduling the second session, a delay that often improves a resident's response to more probing behavioral questions.

Often, the answers people give immediately after admission may be overly influenced by emotion or the residual effects of recent medical treatment. In other words, what they say while trying to adjust to such a new set of circumstances may not be an accurate representation of who they are or how they feel. It is also likely that a resident's orientation and abilities will improve once he or she is medically stabilized, well-nourished, and well-hydrated.

To get an accurate assessment of cognition, sensory skills, and needs and preferences, be sure to pick a private interview location. Privacy will help the resident feel more at ease. Likewise, pick a time of day when the individual is at his or her best. If observation suggests that an individual is more alert in the mornings, schedule a morning interview; if someone seems happier after the day gets underway, schedule something after lunch. In any event, the second session should be accomplished before the first care plan meeting, which is typically scheduled 21 days after admission.

The resident's answers to the behavioral questions provided in this chapter should have a major influence on the final care plan, which must be tailored to the emerging picture of the individual. While the minimum requirement for care plan evaluation is ninety days, I urge you to re-evaluate long before that. Waiting until three months have passed results in nothing so much as missed opportunities – opportunities to ensure that the person-centered care plan is as effective as possible. As you learned from the interventions described in the case studies, effective care plans must be fluid and revised in tandem with the individual's changing needs.

Prepare for a Win-Win Situation

By looking more closely at the individuals in your care, by coming to understand their perspectives on life and living, and by observing how they interact and respond to their current circumstances will do more for you and your team than simply defining a better care plan. It is often just as or more rewarding for a caregiver to crack the code of person-centered care as it is for the resident who receives it. Since there is no universal approach to person-centered care, no cookie-cutter, one-size-fits-all solution, you can take genuine pride in developing interventions that create joy and satisfaction where before there was only despair or fear.

Regulation and policy aside, long-term care is only truly successful when there is a genuine interest in the resident and his or her well-being. You have that interest or you wouldn't be reading the final chapter of this book. You can achieve person-centered care because you now know how to spot the single tree of hope in the great, big forest of frustration.

Good luck!

Made in the USA
Monee, IL
26 October 2022